CROHN'S CRISIS AND CHRISTIANITY

CROHN'S CRISIS AND CHRISTIANITY

LORETTA EASTWOOD

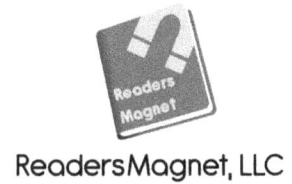

ReadersMagnet, LLC

Crohn's Crisis and Christianity
Copyright © 2020 by Loretta Eastwood

Published in the United States of America
ISBN Paperback: 978-1-953616-43-2
ISBN eBook: 978-1-953616-44-9

All rights reserved. No part of this publication may be reproduced, stored in a retrieval system or transmitted in any way by any means, electronic, mechanical, photocopy, recording or otherwise without the prior permission of the author except as provided by USA copyright law.

KJV
Scripture quotations marked KJV are from the Holy Bible, King James Version (Authorized Version). First published in Quoted from the ICJV Classic Reference Bible.

The opinions expressed by the author are not necessarily those of ReadersMagnet, LLC.

ReadersMagnet, LLC
10620 Treena Street, Suite 230 | San Diego, California, 92131 USA
1.619.354.2643 | www.readersmagnet.com

Book design copyright © 2020 by ReadersMagnet, LLC. All rights reserved.
Cover design by Ericka Obando
Interior design by Renalie Malinao

Contents

Seeing and Meeting My Birth Mother and Father 1
Nieces and Nephew 2
Crohn's Disease 6
Hospital Stays Away from My Son and My Daughter 8
My walk with Crohn's Disease 15
My Job as a Nanny 18
Code of Ethics for Security Guards 19
My Life with My Husband—Our Marriage 21
Adoption of My Daughter 22
My Walk with Crohn's Disease 23
My Inner Thoughts on Crohn's Disease 25
The Church Is a Gift from God 27
Angels 29
Conquering Crohn's 31
My Letters to God 32
A Christmas Letter 35
Prayer for our Nation 38
Top Ten Predictions for 2017 and Beyond 40
Crohn's: Working Through the Pain, Push Yourself 42
Your Decision 45
At the Present Time 47

My purpose for writing this book is to bring awareness to Crohn's disease. I also want people to know it is a crisis—a chronic disease—and to explain my walk and my journey through life.

This book is dedicated to my Lord and Savior Jesus Christ, who walks beside me every minute of the day.

Let me introduce myself. My name is Loretta D Eastwood. I am a sixty-three-year-old white female of Puerto Rican and Italian descent. Growing up, I lived in a foster home in Valhalla, New York, with Jennie Baker, my mom, and Frank Baker, my foster father, whom I am forever grateful for. My foster parents were born in Poland and migrated to the United States, and they spoke fluent Polish to each other. Growing up, I had two foster sisters and four foster brothers.

My childhood was very good. I had a great deal of fun with my brothers and sisters. We played many games, such as baseball, kickball, and dodgeball.

I also remember playing hide-and-seek with the neighbor children and my brothers and sisters until dusk. We also played red rover, red rover; red light, green light; holding hands; and London Bridge and Ring around the Rosie. Hopscotch was in at that time; other games included jump rope, Tag You're It, and spinning around until you were so dizzy you would fall down.

At a young age, I remember the window being left down on summer nights, and I loved to hear the sound of crickets.

Saturday morning we woke up to cereal for breakfast and then watched cartoons.

On hot summer days, we ran through the sprinkler to cool off. I was a bit of a tomboy—I was always climbing trees and riding my bike. At that time, bike riding was not the in thing to do.

We had a swing set; I used to swing so, so high. I loved it when my hair was in the wind. Kool-Aid was a refreshing drink during the summer months. When we all were tired because of playing so hard, I used to take time to lie on the grass and see the beautiful shapes in the clouds.

I must say, nature was a force that governed my life.

At night we would catch fireflies, and that would take up the entire evening. I also loved catching lightning bugs in a jar at night and seeing them light up. Christmas was a very special time growing up. I truly loved Christmas, my best holiday. I loved receiving my presents and going to church and the very beautiful Christmas tree.

We had a very delicious meal—turkey and ham and vegetables and lots of pies and cake. It was so beautiful. Bedtime prayers were a must. My mom and dad were Catholic—I was raised Catholic.

My mom made sure I had my seven sacraments—baptism, Holy Communion, the Eucharist, confirmation, penance, sacraments for the sick, and CCD classes by the nuns. I was even married in the Catholic church.

At the age of six years old, I used to go in the woods by myself and be in solitude for hours, praying and enjoying nature by myself. I called the area in the woods my special place. From time to time, I would see beautiful birds, frogs, squirrels, dogs, snakes, and many different kinds of insects. I was ever grateful for God's creation.

My greatest enjoyment was school. I was on the honor roll till sixth grade. Learning came easy for me. I loved all my teachers. I had several best friends growing up, and I was very loyal to them. My mom was a stay-at-home mom. She was always there when I carne home from school. Before I left for school, I gave my mother a kiss; and when I came home, I gave her another kiss. My mom was my best friend. I spent a great deal of time with her and always enjoyed teatime with her.

I loved to go on field trips at school; that was my favorite, going to museum and different places.

My allowance was a quarter a week. I also helped a neighbor in taking in her groceries, and she paid me fifty cents each time. At that time, at twelve years old, I started babysitting for the neighborhood. I started with my neighbor across the street who had a deaf child. Another mother had two children who were close in age. I helped three times a week with bathing and feeding her children. I loved children.

Then a night, I babysat for a family with five girls. They were all adorable and so good. I also babysat a boy and a girl when I was thirteen. I was very alert. The boy locked himself in the bathroom. I called the mother, and she came home and took care of the situation right away.

All in all, I babysat every summer and became very responsible. At thirteen, I became a candy striper at Grasslands Hospital, and I worked once a week. I knew I was going to pursue a nursing career. I loved working as a candy striper with the nurses at that time. They taught me to take the patients' temperatures.

Seeing and Meeting My Birth Mother and Father

As I said in this book, I used to go out to my secret place in the woods and pray. Being a foster girl, I was always curious in seeing my birth mother. I used to go to the woods and pray to see her. Well, my prayers were answered. Social services sent a social worker to my house, and she asked me to see my birth mother. I was thrilled. I remember I went to a restaurant in white plains, and I was thirteen years old. I had a hamburger and french fries. She explained to me she could not take care of me and did not want me to be mad. I wasn't. I was only happy to see her. She died two months later of heart failure. I was so sad at that time.

Nieces and Nephew

One day I decided to call my niece. She kept the same name as my sisters. I looked her up in the phone book and called her. She lived in Danbury, then she introduced me to her sisters. I then met my nieces, which I am forever grateful.

Then one of my nieces told me about her five-year-old brother. I looked for him and look him up. He lived in Middletown, Upstate New York, and we had a family reunion. He was just about to enter the service.

We met him and had dinner before he entered the service. We went to his wedding. He has four children now, and he still remains in the service. I love him very much, and I am praying to the heavenly Father daily for his protection.

In 1970 I graduated from high school. I applied to a nursing school and was accepted at Grasslands Hospital's LPN program. I passed with an A average. I then received a job at the Grasslands Hospital as a licensed practical nurse. In 1971 I started my job.

In 1975 I got married and moved to Mahopac, New York. My husband had a child from a previous marriage. His first wife died of colitis at Walson Army Hospital.

As I was working on the job, I had episodes of diarrhea. I went to the clinic repeatedly to see the doctor. The first diagnosis said I was malingering. The doctor thought I was there because I was faking it. I also had stomach pains. After a year of repeatedly seeing the doctor, they admitted me and diagnosed me with Crohn's disease (ileitis) sinopsis in 1976.

Crohn's disease is an incurable chronic inflammatory disease of the digestive tract. In fact, Crohn's disease was named after Dr. Burrill B. Crohn, who first described the disease in 1932 along with his colleagues.

Crohn's disease is an inflammatory bowel disorder (IBD) of our own organ. It usually affects the lowest portion of the small intestine (the ileum), but it can occur in other parts of the digestive tract—from the mouth to the anus. Crohn's disease causes inflammation that extends deep into the lining of the intestinal walls, frequently causing cramps, abdominal pain, diarrhea, rectal bleeding, loss of appetite, and weight loss. A common complication of the disease is the blockage of the intestine, which may also occur through the development of scar tissue that narrows the passageway. People with Crohn's disease also suffer from nutritional deficiencies. The disorder affects people in all age groups, but the onset usually occurs between ages fifteen and thirty.

When reading about IBD, it is important to know that Crohn's disease is the same as ulcerative colitis, another type of IBD. The symptoms of these two illnesses are quite similar, but the areas affected in the gastrointestinal tract are different.

They made the diagnosis with a barium x-ray of the small intestine and various biopsies of my small intestine at that time.

In Crohn's disease, the inflammation of the intestine can skip, which means having normal areas in between patches of the diseased intestine, which was exactly what happened to me with my condition.

I had all the symptoms related to Crohn's disease of the GI tract:

- Fever
- Persistent diarrhea
- Rectal bleeding
- Urgent bowel movements
- Abdominal cramps, pain, and vomiting
- Loss of appetite
- Weight loss
- Fatigue
- Night sweats
- Loss of normal menstruation

Treatment at that time involved surgery and heavy steroids.

I experienced loss of appetite and loss of weight, and as a result, I had feelings of low energy and fatigue.

With my Crohn's, it was chronic. I experienced periods when the disease flared up, causing symptoms followed by periods of remission. In my case, I had tears and fissures in the lining of the anus.

Diet and stress may aggravate Crohn's disease, but they do not care for the disease. Recent research suggests hereditary genetics and environmental factors contribute to the development of Crohn's disease.

My disease was caused by environmental factors because I suspect the water system was aged and the pipes were bad. The water was brown at times and corrosive to pipes and plumbing in the house. I saw many people with cancer living in houses around me, and I noticed five people within the block that developed cancer and passed away.

I had my first and only child in 1976. When I was pregnant, they suggested I have an abortion due to my diagnosis of Crohn's disease, but I realized I could not because I thought this might be my only child. My religion, being a Catholic, played an important role. I was totally against abortion. I did not take the doctor's suggestions.

The anointing of the sick is a special sacrament for those who are ill. It is a sign of the healing power of the spirit of Jesus, and its medicinal powers cure the body.

I received the sacrament of the anointing of the sick many times when I was pregnant. I also had a priest lay a hand on my baby in my belly once a month to pray due to my Crohn's crisis at that time. I had a great deal of vomiting. I was getting an iron shot every week and knew the baby was going to be small. At seven months, I went into labor unexpectedly, and I delivered a three-pound-and-two-ounce baby.

My baby was born at Putnam Hospital and then transported to New York Cornell Medical Center. I was in a great deal of prayer at this time because I knew this might be my only child. My son continued to thrive, and after one month of being in the hospital, I took my son home with me. What a blessing the Lord enabled me to have. To this day I call my son the apple of my eye. He now has four children of his own, and they are healthy.

Crohn's Disease

Through the course of my lifetime, I had six surgeries, the last one being in 2005. All my surgeries were end-to-end anastomosis; they cut out one foot of my intestine each time. The doctor always said I had enough intestines left. Also, throughout the course of my lifetime, I had numerous endoscopies to visually examine the interior of my colon.

I also saw numerous doctors throughout my lifetime:

- Gastrointestinal doctor
- Colon and rectal specialist
- Surgeons
- Rheumatologist
- Ophthalmologist
- Gynecologist
- Pain management doctor

I had every area of my body biopsied. I had many rectal biopsies, intestinal biopsies, and vaginal biopsies. At one time I was admitted to the hospital for a 104-degree temperature, and they did a CAT scan and saw a spot on my pancreas and asked me if I could have endoscopy of my pancreas for three years in a row. I also had stomach biopsies to see if I could handle gluten or if I needed a gluten-free diet. I was not allergic to gluten. The only thing in life I cannot tolerate is milk or milk products. I am lactose intolerant.

As of now, I go to a pain doctor. They assess your pain and give you pain medicine. I take pain medications, but I also pray the pain away. Through prayer, you can ask God to help you deal with your pain. I have been in pain throughout my life, and I feel that through the medication and God, I have dealt with it.

The one medication I take for Crohn's disease is Cimzia injections twice a month, 200 mg/mL prefilled syringes, one on the fifteenth of the month and one on the thirtieth every month.

My RN School at Dutchess

After I was working as an LPN at Grasslands Hospital, I decided to go to registered nursing. Even though I had Crohn's in 1980, I went part-time at Dutchess Community College. I took school very seriously. I made sure I received all A on all tests. I did all my readings and did all labs and clinical duties. I never missed a night of school. I went to school in the evening and worked in the day full-time.

I was on the dean's list three times. I went to school part-time for four to five years. I loved to study and learn and further my career. I had help from my husband, my mother, and my mother-in-law and father-in-law in babysitting for my children.

Hospital Stays Away from My Son and My Daughter

I had six surgeries for my Crohn's. I was away a great deal for Christmas and Thanksgiving. My husband, my mother-in-law, and my father-in-law were there for the children while I was admitted. I was truly grateful at that time. I had long hospital stays. Most times it was three weeks to a month. My job would always take me back for work.

At that time, I had hyperalimentation, a special IV therapy and lipids IV, to maintain my weight and give my bowel a rest. I also stayed on prednisone and sulfur—a decreasing dose of prednisone. I was admitted for fever, loss of appetite, weight loss, fatigue, night sweats, and a feeling of low energy.

My disease is chronic, so this means I experience periods when the disease flares up and causes symptoms, followed by periods of remission when I do not notice symptoms at all.

The GI tract contains harmless bacteria that aid in digestion. The immune system usually attacks and kills foreign invaders, such as bacteria or fungi and other microorganisms. In normal circumstances, the harmless bacteria in the intestines are protected from an attack. In people with IBD, these bacteria are mistaken for harmless invaders, and the immune system mounts a response. Cells travel out of the blood and into the intestine and produce an inflammation (a normal immune response). This leads to a chronic inflammation, ulceration, and thickening of the intestinal wall and eventually causes the patient symptoms.

With my Crohn's disease, I worked forty years in nursing. I want to let everyone with Crohn's disease or colitis to go on their life, pick a career you love, and do not let the disease define you. Make yourself as happy as you can. After I retired due to my condition, I was a nanny for children, a job that I loved immensely.

I did not let Crohn's interfere with my traveling. I went to London three times; to Italy, Paris, Hawaii, Canada, and Florida multiple times; and to many cruises. I love to travel and meet people. I love museums, history, and different lands, and I love to see how people live. I traveled a great deal when I was young, and I continue to travel now, but on a lighter scale. I have to have my travels planned and organized, with all my medications available and doctor visits before traveling.

Go places you really want to see and visit—live life to the fullest.

This is my résumé from 1989 to 2003, when I had already over twenty years of nursing experience in diverse settings.

One thing in my nursing career is that I loved my career. I had fun times and serious times.

I was loving to my patients.
I was responsible.
I was empathic.
I was very loyal to my job.
I always learned and thought about my jobs:

- 17 years at Grasslands
- 17 years at a nursing home
- 2 years at another nursing home
- 2 years at another home

I always knew that I could come home to my family, lay my head on my pillow, and sleep well at night because I was good to my patients and enjoyed my job immensely.

LORETTA D. EASTWOOD, RN
PO Box 621
Pauling, NY 12564

Dear Sir or Madam,

I am writing to explore career opportunities as a nanny and/or private nurse for pediatric clients.

During the past two years, I have been employed as a nanny, providing nutrition, hygiene, recreational activities, transportation, and tutoring services. Prior to this position, I worked as a registered nurse in a variety of settings, including skilled nursing, home care, and medical/surgical practice in a hospital environment.

The opportunity to work with children is a very special calling. Those of us who pursue this field are rewarded by the manner in which we enrich the lives of children. In addition, a childcare provider must be a coach, a mentor, and a role model, while building the child's self-esteem and addressing their physical and emotional health. I value a philosophy of caring combined with a personal commitment to performance excellence and continuous improvement.

I have enclosed a copy of my résumé for your review and consideration,

Respectfully,
Enclosure

LORETTA D. EASTWOOD, RN
PO Box 61
Mahopac Falls, NY 10542
(845) 628-8241

SUMMARY/ OBJECTIVE: Over twenty years of nursing experience in diverse settings, including hospital medical-surgical, long-term/skilled care, and home care. Exploring career opportunities where my skills, experience, and commitment to health care excellence can be effectively utilized.

WORK EXPERIENCE:

2003-Present

CORTLANDT HEALTHCARE FACILITY, Cortlandt, NY
REGISTERED NURSE MANAGER, *day position*

- Established a knowledge of MDS's and QA
- Oversaw a staff of professionals requiring excellent leadership and communication skills
- Developed and implemented care plans, working with interdisciplinary team members
- Tracked and monitored patient programs through the continuum of care

SOMERS MANOR, *a long-term/skilled care facility,* Somers, NY
REGISTERED NURSE/CHARGE NURSE

1989-2003

- Supervised nurse's aides in a 100-bed unit
- Participated in treatment planning, from initial patient admission through the entire continuum of care
- Performed discharge planning
- Provided direct patient care including patient documentation/observation, administration of medications, wound care, oxygen therapy, suctioning, range of motion therapy, etc.
- Interfaced with interdisciplinary team members to develop and monitor care plans
- Used interpersonal skills to address the emotional and physical needs of patients
- Coached, mentored, and evaluated nurse's aides
- Selected as preceptor for newly hired employees
- Participated in regulatory adults and JCAHO accreditation

AFFILIATED HOME CARE,
Mahopac, NY
PER DIEM SUPERVISOR

1993-2001
- Supervised a staff of home health aides
- Provided direct patient care in a home setting
- Oversaw patient care provided by home health aides

WESTCHESTER MEDICAL CENTER, Valhalla, NY
<u>**REGISTERED NURSE**</u>, *Medical/Surgical Floor*

1971-1989
- Provided direct patient care in a high traffic medical/surgical floor
- Worked with interdisciplinary team members to develop, monitor, and evaluate treatment plans
- Performed multiple nursing procedures including preop/postop care, IV therapy, oxygen therapy/suctioning, cardio-respiratory assessment/management, pain management, medication administration, crisis intervention, assist with medical procedures, patient education, etc.
- Used interpersonal skills to deal with the emotional needs of patients and family members
- Interfaced with physicians and interdisciplinary team members
- Performed patient admissions and discharge planning
- Started as an LPN and became an RN in 1984

LORETTA EASTWOOD

LICENSE(S):	***Registered Nurse**, State of New York;* ***Licensed Practical Nurse**, State of New York*
EDUCATION:	**WESTCHESTER COMMUNITY COLLEGE** *Pursuing a Bachelor's Degree* in NURSING **DUTCHESS COMMUNITY COLLEGE** *Associates Degree* in MEDICAL SCIENCE **WESTCHESTER COUNTY MEDICAL CENTER** *Completed LPN Nursing Program*

QUALIFICATIONS

- Committed to the highest levels of health care excellence
- Strong advocate of positive change, teamwork, and continuous improvement
- High energy level and ability to manage multiple priorities
- Strong sense of ownership and accountability for assigned tasks
- Use of interpersonal skills to deal with patient and family members in a caring/compassionate manner
  References available upon request

My walk with Crohn's Disease

I was diagnosed at twenty-one with Crohn's disease, and in my perspective, I had struggled but conquered with God's help. Doing a job I loved to do helped me get through my disease by helping sick people. I did not dwell on my condition and did not tell my patients, but I made it through and did not let the disease define me.

By being sensitive in life, things affected me more. I took Princess Diana's death hard, and I also took John Lennon's death hard.

I loved Princess Diana and thought she was a true icon and the people's princess. She was an excellent role model who helped so many people.

I also loved John Lennon, a true artist. I loved the Beatles, and thought they are a true artist too young to die a legend of his own time.

Philippians 4:6 tells us not to worry about anything and instead pray about everything. Tell God your needs, and don't forget to thank him for his answers. If you do this, you will experience

God's peace, which is far more wonderful than the human mind can understand. His peace will keep your thoughts and your hearts quiet and at rest as you trust in Christ Jesus.

Trust in the Lord with all thine heart; and lean not unto thine own understanding.
In all thy ways acknowledge him and he shall direct thy paths. (Proverbs 4:5)

When I married my husband, I started attending the Baptist Church because my father-in-law was a Baptist minister. His church was called Patterson Baptist Church.

I drew closer to God through my father-in-law's preaching. My children were raised Baptist because their grandfather was a Baptist minister. My husband was a firefighter and worked every other day, twenty-four on, twenty-four off.

So many of the days, including every Sunday, I had meals over at their place and had devotions with my in-laws and my children and their grandfather. I was very close to my husband's father and loved his preaching. He taught me the Bible very well, and I definitely became closer to God.

My son, my daughter, my husband, and I adored my father-in-law—a truly very special role model, with an unconditional love for all. At present, he is with our Lord and Savior in heaven.

I have been through bad times and good times with my condition. But each time, I used prayer to get through my time. My pain drew me closer to God. I just want to put it out there: If you need to use prayer or a doctor or psychiatrist, use them all. But with Crohn's and colitis, you need a very strong support system.

My husband and I and my children went on vacations a great deal. We took our children to Florida, camping in Maine, and various other parks to picnic. On the holidays, we went to various parties.

I had a very close girlfriend who was truly there for me all the time. She came in the hospital, visited me and comforted me all the time. She was very supportive and helped me get through many surgeries. We worked together for many years, and I was at her house for many meals. I am forever grateful for her. God bless her.

My husband and God were truly my rock and support throughout my surgeries and recovery. My husband was very proud of me. He sent me flowers many times. He also brought me lunch sometimes on his days off. I used to really enjoy that, and through the years, he brought me jewelry of all kinds—rings, necklaces, and bracelets. I really enjoyed those precious moments and will always remember them.

My Job as a Nanny

My doctor encouraged me to retire and go on disability. I really missed my nursing career. I was very upset but decided to go on disability. I remember crying at the disability office. I went on to be a nanny. At this time, I love children. I babysat for a child with a closed nare (nose). She had two surgeries, and she needed medicine and nebulizer treatments. She also had a sister. I was also a nanny for another lady for her baby, four months old till five, and she also had a set of twins I started babysitting at four months old. I loved all the children I babysat for. I also tutored the children and taught all of them with flash cards and math books. Another nanny job was for a lady who had two children, a boy and a girl, whom I cherished very much.

I always loved all the children and always thought they were a true blessing from God. At the same time, I went for armed security guard—just for training and backup. I wanted training. I never worked as a security guard, but just went for the training with my husband and passed my armed guard course.

Code of Ethics for Security Guards

In my capacity as a security guard, hired to prevent, report, and deter crime, I pledge

- A. to protect life and property, prevent and reduce crime committed against my employer/client's business or other organizations and institutions to which I am assigned, abide by the Constitution of the United States;
- B. to carry out my duties with honesty and integrity and to maintain the highest moral principles;
- C. to faithfully, diligently, and dependably discharge my duties, and to uphold the laws, policies, and procedures that protect the rights of others;
- D. to discharge my duties truthfully, accurately, and prudently without interference of personal feelings, prejudices, animosities, or friendships to influence my judgments;
- E. to report any violation of law or rule or regulation immediately to my superiors;

F. to respect and protect information considered confidential and privileged by my employer or client, except where their interests are contrary to law or this Code of Ethics;
G. to cooperate with all recognized and responsible law enforcement agencies within their jurisdiction;
H. to accept no compensation, commission, gratuity, or other advantage without the knowledge and consent of my employer;
I. to conduct myself professionally at all times and to perform my duties in a manner that reflects credit upon myself, my employer, and the security profession;
J. to continually improve my performance by seeking training and educational opportunities that better prepare me to carry out my security duties.

When my husband's mother, Helen, was well, we lived side by side in a mother-daughter home. We took her on many vacations to Rhode Island, Boston, Mystic, Connecticut, and many family functions. My husband's mother was diagnosed with Alzheimer's at seventy-two, and we moved her from Mahopac to Pawling, in our home. We took care of her for thirteen years with her sickness. My husband was very good in taking care of his mother with me. We did it as long as we could.

In 2012, my husband decided to move from New York to South Carolina to be nearer to our daughter. It was hard for me to make the transition to South Carolina and to get a new set of doctors. The ride to South Carolina was not a good ride—I was in pain. I was told when I came down, they were going to do surgery. But when I was examined, they changed their minds. I went to a hospital MUSC, and they examined me more under anesthesia and I seemed to be doing somewhat better.

My Life with My Husband—Our Marriage

I was introduced to my husband on a blind date. We dated for one year and then married. When I married my husband, his daughter was three years old. He worked as a firefighter—twenty-four hours on, twenty-four hours off. I worked full-time as a nurse. We had very busy schedules. My husband was in the Air National Guard. I did go to London for a month with him.

We both worked hard through the years. We enjoyed many vacations together. My husband did attend many of my doctor visits with me, which I am grateful for.

Adoption of My Daughter

When I was married in 1975 to my husband, he had a three-year-old daughter. So I was an immediate mother to his little girl. She was a beautiful blond girl, and I always loved fixing her hair and dressing her up on holidays.

My daughter now is living with her husband in South Carolina and has two children.

As I raised up my children, and are with my grandchildren.

The most important thing in life is not the kind of cars they own or the job they have or how much money they have. I am happy to say that the most important thing is to know Jesus Christ as their personal Lord and Savior.

My Walk with Crohn's Disease

I was diagnosed at twenty-one with Crohn's disease, and in my perspective, I had a struggled but conquered with God's help. Doing a job I loved to do helped me get through my disease, by helping sick people. I did not dwell on my condition and did not tell my patients, but I made it through.

By being sensitive in life, things affected me more. I took Princess Diana's death hard, and I also took John Lennon's death hard.

I loved Princess Diana and thought she was a true icon and the people's princess. She was an excellent role model who helped so many people. I also loved John Lennon, a true artist. I also loved the Beatles and thought they are a true artist too young to die, a legend of his own time.

I loved nature and God's creation. The woods in the backyard where I lived in Valhalla were the best thing. I loved to play in the woods, sit and think, and just observe.

I always relied on God mostly due to my disease and working with the disease. It made me look at life differently, made me not to take things for granted and to be ever grateful for everything.

With Crohn's disease, I was very tired. I had fatigue. I napped and slept well.

I loved Sundays—going to church and having breakfast at my man's house. We had bacon and eggs and roast beef dinner at night. Life was good.

My Inner Thoughts on Crohn's Disease

Life is forever changing—go with the changes.
Always have fun in life.
All things are possible with God's help.
Take your challenges and go through them full speed ahead.
Dwell on your strengths.
Be kind to yourself.
Love yourself.
Life is a learning experience.
Count your blessings.
Always stay positive in life.
Have fun in life- live, love, and laugh.
There is always something to be thankful for.
Being happy in life helps with any condition—everyone deserves to be happy.
Try not to feel stressed—do something to decrease stress.
Appreciate the fine things and the small things in life.
Love nature and God's creation.

If bored, do something; do something unexpected. Be spontaneous. Take a risk for once.
Be grateful for the small things.

Sending love and hugs to all. God bless all!

My father-in-law was the head pastor of Have fun in life—Paterson Baptist Church in New York. I felt a deep connection with my father-in-law. He displayed unconditional love throughout his lifetime to everyone. I attended church regularly with him along with my son and daughter.

When I wasn't able to go to church due to my job as a nurse, he would drive the children to church. Because they were around their grandparents a great deal of time, the children became born-again Christians, and they attended Baptist Church.

The one goal in life I achieved was to make sure my children were Christians and attended church every Sunday. At this time, they are raising their children the same way.

The Church Is a Gift from God

Well, as I look on God, he gives us gifts in life. Coming down here at the age sixty-two was a challenge for me.

The reality is that I felt somewhat disconnected from churches, my family, and friends. I loved my family, my husband's family, and my churches.

But truly, God gives gifts. I am very blessed with the churches here where I live so I can learn the Word and draw nearer to God. I always ask for God's divine intervention and prayer for me. As I greet people for a handshake, I always say, "God bless," and in prayer, I always, deep inside, want God to pour out his blessing on each and every person. My prayer for all is to always find peace and comfort from our Heavenly Father and for him to pour out his blessing on all. From time to time in my life, I know God has shown us. They regard our safety, undertake our me signs and given me spiritual, divine defenses, and direct our ways, and they exercise intervention. a constant solicitude that no evil befalls on us.

Doves are special in my life. He sent doves for me to see, and I definitely knew he was speaking to me, saying everything was all right. Two times he sent to me two praying mantises, which I gazed upon for hours. One was so big I ended up petting it, and I quietly said, "Thank you, Heavenly Father."

When I was sick with Crohn's crises, I had my baby blessed and prayed on, and I knew God had his hand in making my journey and giving the doctor knowledge at that time to have my baby live and grow stronger every day. One time I even thought God showed me divine intervention through a statue of Jesus, Mary, and Joseph.

The angels are the dispersers and administrators of the divine beneficence toward us. They regard our safety, undertake our defenses, and direct our ways, and they exercise a constant solicitude that no evil befalls on us.

Angels

I had a garage sale and had a statue my mother gave me of Jesus, Mary, and Joseph. It had many chips and cracks on it. A man in a black car came to me and asked for the statue, and I said, "Sir, my mother gave this statue to me. My husband put it here on mistake."

The man picked up the statue and said, "I really want it."

I replied, "Sir, take anything on the table for free. I am so sorry my husband put it out, and it was a mistake."

So I asked him why he was so interested in the statue. He replied to me, "See all those chips in the statue? I want as many blessings as you have in the statue. That is why I want the statue."

I knew right away God sent this man to me with divine intervention to say, "Know you are blessed due to the chips in the statue."

Whenever I go away traveling and I see a church, I stop and say a prayer to God and have prayer time.

I also had the blessing of the Holy Spirit coming into me at a church in New York. It was a whole day of prayer, and if one ever experiences it, you will know the Holy Spirit has come inside you immediately. You can definitely feel the presence of the Holy Spirit. After the entire experience, I stayed in the church an extra two hours of silent prayer for this intervention from God.

My greatest joy is walking by the beach as I silently pray to God all prayers during my walk. I can scarcely take all the magnificent look of God's creation, constantly look at the majestic sea, and pray without ceasing.

Yes, I love talking and being in communion with our Heavenly Father. Prayer has definitely changed so much in my life, and I even say to my grandchildren that I am leaving them with a legacy of prayer—the greatest gift I can leave them.

I am blessed with the pastors in church. I go to two churches now, and church is the greatest thing in life. I love all pastors preaching. I learn something every time they preach the Word of God, and I can tell at this time, I am closer to God. Once in a while at the church I attend, I eat lunch with the pastor. They knew and loved my father-in-law. I feel so blessed in my life to know all my pastors and to experience their unconditional love for God and their deep compassion.

Lord, let my eyes see what your eyes see, like flood your being.

Conquering Crohn's

I must say I relied on God throughout my years. I prayed and I still do. Right now, I live in South Carolina, the Bible Belt. I go to church usually two times, on Sunday and Wednesday night. If we don't go on Wednesday night, we have Bible devotions in the morning. I read the Bible or other books with Bible verses called devotional books. I also write letters to Jesus. I have written twenty-five letters, which I love.

Here are ten of the letters to help me with my Crohn's disease. I wrote letters to God for peace and comfort and to help me deal with my condition. I wrote a total of twenty-five, but here are just a few.

My Letters to God

A NOTE TO GOD

Dear Heavenly Father,

Thank you for the many blessings you bestowed on me. Dear Heavenly Father, thank you for your promise to bring us to victory. I ask for your strength as I take a stand to do what is right according to your Word. I know your hand of blessing is upon our every acts of obedience. I bless your name today, and I will seek to serve you in everything I do.

With much love,
Loretta D. Eastwood

Dear Heavenly Father,

Thank you for your hand of blessing on our life today. I purpose in my heart to raise my level of expectancy and hope in you. Thank you for putting your desires in my heart and bringing them to pass in my life.

Dear Heavenly Father, thank you for being my defender. I ask you right now to search my heart and show me anything that appears that I have not released to you. Help me forgive those who have wronged me so that I may be free to live in victory.

Love,
Loretta D. Eastwood

Dear Jesus, Lord, Messiah, Abba, _Alpha. Omega,

Happy Thanksgiving!
I received a card in the mail saying, "What are you thankful for?"
I am thankful for family, love, home, laughter, and friends. I am thankful for the privilege of you protecting me. And thank you for the Bible.
John 3:16: "For God so loved the world that he gave his only begotten son that whosoever believeth in him should not perish but have everlasting life."
Heaven equals total bliss.

Loretta D. Eastwood

Dear Jesus,

    I have so much to be thankful for, so I ask you as the Bible says in Psalm 19:14, "Let the words of my mouth and the meditations of my heart be acceptable in thy sight. 0 Lord, my strength and my redeemer."

    I want to thank you for showing me signs from heaven in your own way. As I praise and worship during the day, I see signs that you comfort me, and then I say, "Yes, that is Jesus giving me another sign of comfort."

    I am thankful for the moment. I am also thankful for my foundation in you. I am reassured with Psalm 62:7-8:

> In God is my salvation and my glory.
> The rock of my strength and my refuge is in God.
> Trust in him at all times, ye people.
> Pour out your heart before him.
> God is a refuge for us Selah, Amen.

Loretta D. Eastwood

A Christmas Letter

As we say "Merry Christmas," this is an expression of joy and hope represented by the birth of Christ. It is the time for celebrating the greatest gift ever shared: the birth of Christ.

"Today in the town of David, a Savior has been born to you. He is Christ the Lord."

I look to you as my mentors and my friends. Peace and Jesus's love and his embrace to you, and I leave you with these words:

> Jesus spoke saying, "I am the light of the world—whoever follows me will not walk in darkness but will have the light of life." (John 8:12)

Dear Friends in Christ
Dear Jesus
a letter of love and faith by Loretta D. Eastwood

God promises to give us everything we need to walk according to his will. God expects us and delights in us to walk according to his will.

God expects us and delights in us to walk:
To walk in the newness of life
To walk according to his Holy Spirit
To walk in honesty
To walk in faith, not by sight
To walk in good works
To walk according to the Holy Spirit
To walk worthy of his calling
To walk in Jesus Christ
To walk in love
To walk as children of the Light
To walk circumspectly
To walk in wisdom
To walk in a manner that praises him
To walk in truth
To walk worthy of him
To walk according to his commandments
To walk in fear of the Lord

The ability to demonstrate these qualities in life is found in the promise of God.

Rejoice in the Lord always, rejoice. Let your gentleness be evident. The lord is near. Do not be anxious about anything, but in everything by prayer and petition with thanksgiving, present your requests to God. (Philippians 4:4-6)

In conclusion, everyone should be encouraged by God to grant themselves forgiveness for their failings and not live in fear and guilt, but always keep on trying to live a grander vision of what

God wants for all of us. God does not expect more from you than what he promises to provide for you. His strength and righteous power and love, wisdom and truth are part and parcel of his special promises to you.

Trust his promises, and then try your best and leave the rest to God.

Note to God

Dear friends in Christ,
Dear Jesus,

This is a letter of love and faith and thankfulness. Thank you, Jesus, for your promise that gives us everything we need to walk according to your will. Thank you for giving us grace and delighting in us when we walk. Thank you for helping us walk in the newness of life.

Dear Jesus Lord, please make my house a home of prayer and peace. Thank you in advance. Everyone's house should serve as a house of prayer for our family and friends. Upon entering the house, the Spirit of the Lord should be obvious. Please make my house peaceful. The Christian house may be quiet; the Holy Spirit's presence should be obvious.

Thank you, Lord. Lord, please make my house yours. Please make my house a house of prayer—a place of peace and comfort, a refuge to those in need. And in conclusion, help me make our house a blessing for all who pass through the door. Thank you, Lord.

Joshua 24:15: "As for me and my house, we will serve the Lord."

Prayer for our Nation

Almighty God, you have given us this great nation as our heritage.

We humbly pray that we may always remember your generosity and faithfully do your will. Bless our land and nation with honest industry, truthful education, and an honorable way of life.

Defend our liberties and strengthen the resolve of the people who have come from throughout the world to make America their home. Lead us to choose the harder right instead of the easier wrong. Help us to appreciate the opportunities that are ours as we struggle to bring harmony to an unsettled world.

May we balance our concern for prejudice with a willingness to display mercy, and may our concern for security be tempered with a willingness to take risks, which will produce worthwhile changes for the good of all people. O Lord, we pray for guidance as we work together for the best interest of our communities, our nation, our world, and the ultimate goal of peace.

When times are prosperous, let our hearts be thankful, and in troubled times, may our deepest trust be in you. Amen.

Those who hope in the Lord will renew their strength They will soar on wings like eagles They will run and not grow weary They will walk and not be faint (Isaiah 40:31)

Oh Heavenly Father Look down from heaven and see We will not turn away from you Receive us and we will call your name. Make your face shine upon us That we may be saved (Psalm 80:14, 18-19)

Top Ten Predictions for 2017 and Beyond

The Bible will still have all the answers.
Prayer will still be the most powerful thing on earth.
The Holy Spirit will still move. God will still honor the praises of his people.
There will still be God in anointed preaching.
There will still be singing of praise to God.
God will still pour out blessings upon his people.
There will still be room at the cross.
Jesus will always love you.

Jesus will still save the lost when they come to him. Isn't it great to remember who is really in control and that the "word of the Lord endures forever" (1 Peter 1:25)?

Just remember, problems are a part of everyone's life. Do not tend to go to solving everyone's problem. You have to always remind yourself that you do not have the capacity to fix everyone's problems, just your immediate family's problems. Also, I always tell people you are number 1; you are top priority. You come first.

Do not take the world's responsibilities on to yourself. Make you relationship with God and your family your primary concern.

In my life, I had to pace myself as an LPN. I worked seven-to-three, came home to two children, cooked dinner, put them to bed, and worked full-time. I was in my twenties. In my forties, I then went to RN School.

I worked full-time and went to school with a part-time schedule and tended to my children. I had help from my mother, my mother-in-law, my husband, and my father-in-law. I needed all the help I could get. I also cleared my house on my days off.

One also has to nurture the body. On my days off, I did relaxing techniques with myself. You should practice relaxation on a daily basis. It helps your relationship with your husband and your children. Relaxation gives you peace of mind and happiness, and it helps you manage stress in your life.

Crohn's: Working Through the Pain, Push Yourself

I learned very early on, living with a condition or disease, that your greatest joy in life is reaching your full potential—be all that you can be.

I experienced some of the most painful and difficult times of my life, and I just strived through them. You go through the process, and you also know you have to push yourself—one foot in front of the other—to reach your outcome. Leave yourself with the independence left within yourself so you can deal with any hardships or troubles. Strive through your full potential. It will help you deal with your adversity.

When you are in your job, do not worry about promotions, for I worked in a job ten years without a promotion. You will never reach your full potential as long as you look at your circumstances and have "I can't" in your vocabulary.

To decrease stress with Crohn's in your life, you have to come to a point in your life where you have to say to yourself, "This problem is too great for me let go!"

Do not handle stress on your shoulders. I will say I found out that with the disease, people have found me weak. I had myself in many situations not fighting or quarreling, just walking away. There was name-calling, and I just walked away. I tried not to let people get the best of me.

At times, you deal with depression. Many times, the doctor offered me antidepressants. I just refused and went to church. You must be strong. Take full control of your life and your circumstances.

There were times in my life when I thought my tasks as a mother, nurse, wife—all the tasks —appeared too great for me to handle. I just strived through and pushed myself.

When everything feels like it's weighing you down, seek positive people for your support system, and never give up hope. Everything boils down to a matter of support and people to trust with all your immediate circumstances.

My husband was my greatest supporter. My best girlfriend was also a huge supporter. My father-in-law was a preacher and was my true supporter, and my sister also gave me great support and help. If you also have God in your life, all things are possible.

Bible quote:
In spite of the struggles, difficulty, sin, or other obstacles that you may have faced, God still has a fantastic plan in mind for your life. This is his personal promise for you.

It is God's plan to give you hope and a future, and his goal is to lead you through the difficult times so that you will fulfill his purpose in your life.

As of now, I am a retired registered nurse living in South Carolina. In my spare time, I go online and have prayers with people who ask me. I answer questions and give my input to people.

At this time, our world is ever changing and is in crisis. I have prayer time with a just deal of people and my contacts.
    Be of strong mind.
    Stay positive.
    Keep laughter and love in your life.
    And thaw closer to God.

Loretta D. Eastwood

> My gift for you is for you to have salvation.
> The way of salvation is through Jesus Christ.
> Romans 5:8-11

But God commandeth his love toward us, in that while we were yet sinners, Christ died for us. Much more then, being now justified by his blood, we shall be saved from wrath through him. For if when we were enemies we were reconciled, we shall be saved by his life, and not only so, but we also rejoice in God through our Lord Jesus Christ, by whom we have now received the atonement.

Your Decision

I now put my faith and trust in Jesus Christ alone as my personal Savior. Believing that Jesus Christ is the Son of God, I acknowledge that I am a sinner and believe that Jesus provides the way of salvation for all those who are willing to come to him for forgiveness. I do now confess him as my Lord and Savior.

This is called the method of receiving God's gift of salvation:

That if thou shalt confess with thy mouth the Lord Jesus, and shalt believe in their heart that God hath raised him from the dead, thou shalt be saved. For with the heart man believeth unto righteousness; and with the mouth confession is made unto salvation. For whosoever shall call upon the name of the Lord shall be saved. (Romans 10:9— 10, 13)

To all who receive him and to those who believe in his name, he gives the right for you to become children of God. You can experience this today if you will ask Christ to come into your heart by faith.

In conclusion, I can help you make your personal commitment to Jesus Christ. Do you trust him alone for your salvation?

I am asking you to please take the step of faith if you are unsure about your relationship with Jesus Christ. Turn to Jesus Christ today and receive him as your personal Lord and Savior. The inner sanctuary of God's throne is always open to those who have repented of sin and trusted Christ as their Savior.

At the Present Time

Heavenly Father,

Our world is in crisis. Lives have been taken, families are grieving, and our hearts are broken. Help us, Holy Father, to draw near to you, to find our hope in Jesus, to pray fervently, and to seek your mercy for all. We need you in a great way, Lord, and we call on you to be in our midst. In these and all things, we pray in Jesus's name. Amen!

In ending this memoir, my conclusion is, I am not a citizen of this world trying to get to heaven. I am a citizen of heaven making my way through this world.

This is my temporary home!

www.ingramcontent.com/pod-product-compliance
Lightning Source LLC
LaVergne TN
LVHW020438080526
838202LV00055B/5256